DIABETES DIET FOR NEWLY DIAGNOSED

Mary Dixon

TABLE OF CONTENT

CHAPTER ONE

Types, Causes and Symptoms of Diabetes

Diabetes is a chronic medical condition that affects how your body regulates blood sugar, also known as glucose. Glucose is a vital source of energy for your cells, and its levels need to be carefully controlled.

When the body cannot maintain normal blood sugar levels, it can lead to diabetes. There are several types of diabetes, each with its own causes and symptoms. In this overview, we'll discuss the main types of diabetes, their causes, and common symptoms.

Types of Diabetes:

1. Type 1 Diabetes:

- Cause: Type 1 diabetes is an autoimmune condition where the immune system mistakenly attacks and destroys insulin-producing beta cells in the pancreas. The exact cause is not fully understood, but it is believed to involve genetic and environmental factors.

- Symptoms: Rapid onset of symptoms, including excessive thirst, frequent urination, unexplained weight loss, fatigue, and blurred vision. It often develops in children and young adults.

2. Type 2 Diabetes:

- Cause: Type 2 diabetes is primarily caused by a combination of genetic predisposition and lifestyle factors such as obesity, poor diet, lack of physical activity, and insulin resistance. Insulin resistance means the body's cells don't respond effectively to insulin.

- Symptoms: Gradual onset of symptoms, including increased thirst, frequent urination, fatigue, blurred vision, slow wound healing, and recurring infections. It typically develops in adulthood but can occur in children and adolescents due to rising obesity rates.

3. Gestational Diabetes:

- Cause: Gestational diabetes occurs during pregnancy when the body cannot produce enough insulin to meet increased insulin demands. Hormonal changes during pregnancy can contribute to insulin resistance.

- Symptoms: Often asymptomatic, but some women may experience increased thirst, frequent urination, and fatigue. Gestational diabetes usually resolves after childbirth, but affected individuals have a higher risk of developing Type 2 diabetes later in life.

Less Common Types of Diabetes:

4. Monogenic Diabetes: Caused by mutations in a single gene, leading to impaired insulin production or function. These cases are often diagnosed in childhood or young adulthood.

5. Secondary Diabetes: Results from another medical condition or the use of certain medications that affect insulin production or action. Examples include pancreatic diseases, hormonal disorders, and the use of corticosteroids.

6. Other Specific Types: This category includes rare forms of diabetes with distinct causes, such as genetic syndromes, infections, or drug-induced diabetes.

Common Symptoms of Diabetes:

- Excessive Thirst (Polydipsia): Increased sugar levels in the blood lead to dehydration, causing intense thirst.
- Frequent Urination (Polyuria): Excess glucose in the bloodstream leads to increased urine production.

- Unexplained Weight Loss: Despite increased appetite, individuals with diabetes may lose weight due to inefficient glucose utilization.
- Fatigue: Cells are deprived of glucose, resulting in low energy levels.
- Blurred Vision: High blood sugar levels can affect the lens in the eye, causing temporary vision problems.
- Slow Wound Healing: Elevated blood sugar impairs the body's ability to heal wounds, increasing the risk of infections.
- Recurrent Infections: High sugar levels can weaken the immune system, making individuals more susceptible to infections.

It's crucial to diagnose and manage diabetes promptly to prevent complications such as heart disease, kidney damage, nerve problems, and vision loss.

Treatment often involves lifestyle modifications, medication, insulin therapy, or a combination of these approaches, depending on the type and severity of diabetes. Regular monitoring and medical care are essential for effectively managing diabetes and maintaining a high quality of life.

Diabetes Diet for Newly Diagnosed and Benefits

Following a diabetes diet is crucial for managing blood sugar levels and overall health for individuals who have been newly diagnosed with diabetes.

A well-balanced diabetes diet can offer several benefits, including better blood sugar control, weight management, and a reduced risk of complications. Here are some guidelines to help you follow a diabetes-friendly diet and reap its benefits:

1. Consult a Registered Dietitian: Upon diagnosis, it's essential to seek guidance from a registered dietitian or healthcare professional who specializes in diabetes. They can help create a personalized meal plan tailored to your specific needs, preferences, and lifestyle.

2. Understand Carbohydrates: Carbohydrates have the most significant impact on blood sugar levels. Learn to count carbohydrates to manage your intake effectively. Focus on complex carbohydrates like whole grains, vegetables, legumes, and fruits, as they provide more stable blood sugar control.

3. Portion Control: Be mindful of portion sizes to avoid overeating and control calorie intake. Measuring your food and using portion control tools can be helpful.

4. Choose Balanced Meals:

- Protein: Include lean protein sources like poultry, fish, tofu, beans, and low-fat dairy in your meals. Protein helps stabilize blood sugar levels and keeps you feeling full.
- Fiber: Fiber-rich foods like vegetables, fruits, whole grains, and legumes can help slow the absorption of carbohydrates and improve blood sugar control.
- Healthy Fats: Incorporate sources of healthy fats like avocados, nuts, seeds, and olive oil. These fats are beneficial for heart health and can help control blood sugar.

5. Limit Added Sugars: Minimize or eliminate sugary foods and beverages from your diet, as they can cause rapid spikes in blood sugar. Read food labels to identify hidden sources of sugar.

6. Monitor Your Blood Sugar: Regularly check your blood sugar levels as recommended by your healthcare provider. This information can help you make necessary adjustments to your diet and medications.

7. Plan Meals: Plan your meals and snacks in advance to maintain consistency in your eating habits. Skipping meals can lead to erratic blood sugar levels.

8. Stay Hydrated: Drink plenty of water throughout the day to stay hydrated. Avoid sugary drinks and excessive caffeine.

9. Be Mindful of Alcohol: If you choose to consume alcohol, do so in moderation and with food. Alcohol can affect blood sugar levels and interact with medications.

10. Regular Physical Activity: Combine your dietary efforts with regular physical activity. Exercise helps improve insulin sensitivity and overall health.

11. Gradual Changes: It may be overwhelming to make significant dietary changes all at once. Start by making small, manageable adjustments and gradually build healthier habits over time.

12. Monitor Progress: Keep track of your meals, blood sugar levels, and how you feel after eating to identify patterns and make necessary adjustments to your diet plan.

13. Regular Follow-Ups: Continually work with your healthcare team to assess your progress and make necessary adjustments to your meal plan and medications.

A diabetes diet can significantly improve your health and quality of life by helping you maintain stable blood sugar levels and reduce the risk of complications.

Remember that it's essential to work closely with your healthcare provider and dietitian to develop a personalized plan that suits your specific needs and goals.

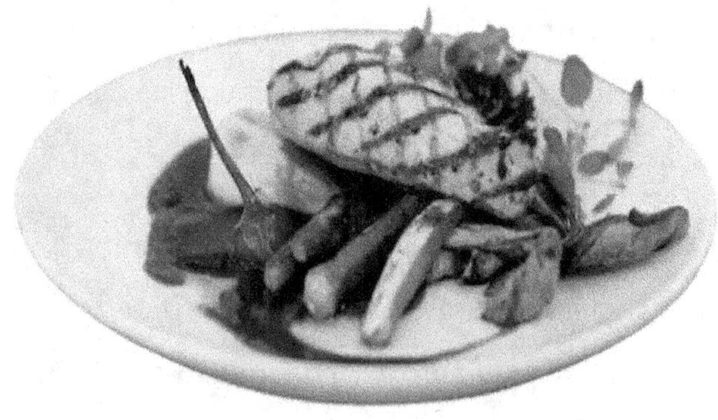

CHAPTER TWO

14-Day Diabetes Diet Meal Plan for Newly Diagnosed

This 14-day diabetes diet meal plan is for someone who is newly diagnosed with diabetes. Please note that individual dietary needs may vary, so it's essential to consult with a registered dietitian or healthcare professional for a personalized plan.

This meal plan provides a general guideline for balanced, diabetes-friendly meals.

Day 1:

- Breakfast: Scrambled eggs with spinach and whole-grain toast.
- Lunch: Grilled chicken breast salad with mixed greens and vinaigrette dressing.
- Snack: Greek yogurt with berries.
- Dinner: Baked salmon with steamed broccoli and quinoa.

Day 2:

- Breakfast: Oatmeal with sliced almonds and a sprinkle of cinnamon.
- Lunch: Turkey and avocado whole-grain wrap with a side of raw veggies.
- Snack: Carrot and cucumber sticks with hummus.
- Dinner: Stir-fried tofu with mixed vegetables and brown rice.

Day 3:

- Breakfast: Cottage cheese with sliced peaches and a drizzle of honey.
- Lunch: Lentil soup with a side of mixed greens and whole-grain crackers.
- Snack: Apple slices with a small portion of peanut butter.
- Dinner: Grilled shrimp with roasted asparagus and quinoa.

Day 4:

- Breakfast: Greek yogurt parfait with granola and fresh berries.

- Lunch: Quinoa and black bean salad with diced tomatoes and lime dressing.

- Snack: A handful of mixed nuts.

- Dinner: Baked chicken breast with steamed green beans and sweet potato.

Day 5:

- Breakfast: Whole-grain waffle topped with almond butter and banana slices.

- Lunch: Spinach and feta stuffed chicken breast with a side of roasted Brussels sprouts.

- Snack: Celery sticks with cream cheese.

- Dinner: Grilled tilapia with sautéed spinach and quinoa.

Day 6:

- Breakfast: Veggie omelette with a side of mixed fruit.
- Lunch: Tuna salad with chickpeas, cucumber, and cherry tomatoes.
- Snack: Sliced bell peppers with guacamole.
- Dinner: Lean beef stir-fry with broccoli and brown rice.

Day 7:

- Breakfast: Smoothie with unsweetened almond milk, spinach, berries, and protein powder.
- Lunch: Whole-grain pasta with marinara sauce and a side of steamed broccoli.
- Snack: Plain popcorn (no butter or added salt).
- Dinner: Baked cod with sautéed spinach and quinoa.

Day 8:

- Breakfast: Scrambled eggs with diced bell peppers and a slice of whole-grain toast.
- Lunch: Turkey and vegetable stir-fry with brown rice.
- Snack: Cottage cheese with pineapple chunks.
- Dinner: Grilled chicken breast with roasted Brussels sprouts and quinoa.

Day 9:

- Breakfast: Whole-grain cereal with low-fat milk and sliced strawberries.
- Lunch: Spinach and mushroom omelette with a side salad.
- Snack: Sliced cucumbers with tzatziki sauce.
- Dinner: Baked salmon with steamed asparagus and brown rice.

Day 10:

- Breakfast: Smoothie with kale, banana, unsweetened yogurt, and a touch of honey.
- Lunch: Lentil and vegetable curry with a side of whole-grain naan bread.
- Snack: A small handful of cherry tomatoes with mozzarella cheese.
- Dinner: Grilled shrimp and vegetable kebabs with quinoa.

Day 11:

- Breakfast: Whole-grain pancakes topped with fresh berries and a dollop of Greek yogurt.
- Lunch: Chicken and vegetable soup with a side of mixed greens.
- Snack: Sliced apple with a sprinkle of cinnamon.
- Dinner: Baked tofu with broccoli and a side of brown rice.

Day 12:

- Breakfast: Scrambled egg whites with spinach and a whole-grain English muffin.
- Lunch: Quinoa salad with roasted vegetables and a balsamic vinaigrette.
- Snack: Celery sticks with almond butter.
- Dinner: Grilled tilapia with lemon and dill, served with sautéed kale and quinoa.

Day 13:

- Breakfast: Cottage cheese and pineapple parfait with a drizzle of honey.

- Lunch: Turkey and avocado lettuce wraps with a side of carrot sticks.

- Snack: Mixed nuts and dried fruit (in moderation).

- Dinner: Lean beef and vegetable stir-fry with brown rice.

Day 14:

- Breakfast: Veggie-packed omelette with a side of mixed fruit.
- Lunch: Whole-grain pasta with pesto sauce and a side of steamed broccoli.
- Snack: Raw bell pepper strips with hummus.
- Dinner: Baked cod with a side of sautéed spinach and quinoa.

Remember to continue monitoring your blood sugar levels, staying hydrated, and engaging in regular physical activity. Adjust your portion sizes and meal choices as needed to maintain stable blood sugar levels, and consult with your healthcare team for ongoing support in managing your diabetes. A balanced and diabetes-friendly diet, like the one outlined here, can help you lead a healthier and more controlled life with diabetes.

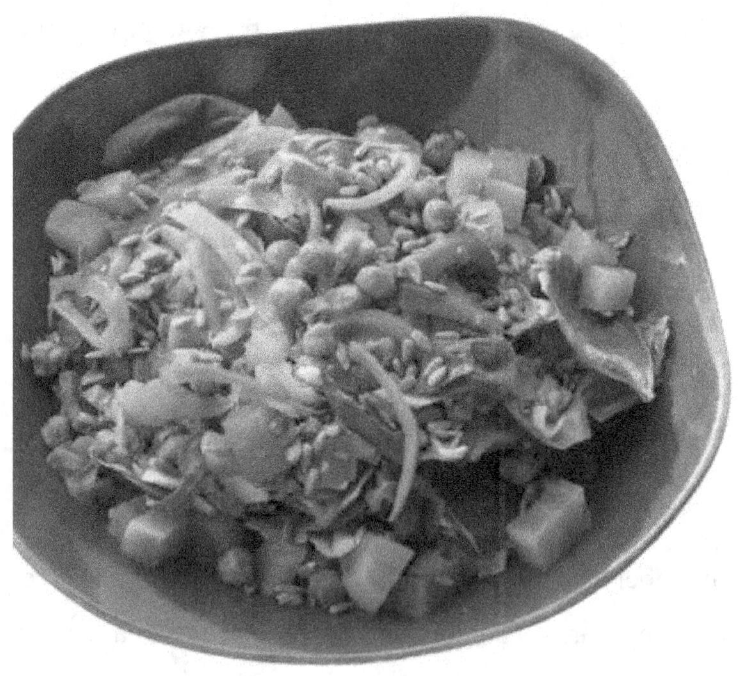

CHAPTER THREE

Diabetes Diet Breakfast Recipes for Newly Diagnosed

These recipes are balanced to help manage blood sugar levels and provide you with a nutritious start to your day. Each recipe includes a short, ingredients, instructions, and estimated cooking time.

1. Veggie Omelette

Start your day with a protein-packed veggie omelette that's low in carbs and rich in nutrients.

Ingredients:

- 2 large eggs
- 1/4 cup diced bell peppers
- 1/4 cup diced onions
- 1/4 cup chopped spinach
- Salt and pepper to taste
- 1 tsp olive oil

Instructions:

1. Whisk eggs in a bowl and season with salt and pepper.

2. Heat olive oil in a non-stick pan over medium heat.

3. Add onions, bell peppers, and spinach. Sauté until tender.

4. Pour whisked eggs into the pan and cook until set.

5. Fold the omelette in half and serve hot.

Cooking Time: Approximately 10 minutes.

2. Greek Yogurt Parfait

This Greek yogurt parfait is a quick and delicious way to incorporate protein and fiber into your breakfast.

Ingredients:

- 1/2 cup Greek yogurt (unsweetened)
- 1/4 cup mixed berries (e.g., strawberries, blueberries)
- 2 tbsp chopped nuts (e.g., almonds, walnuts)
- 1 tsp honey (optional)

Instructions:

1. Layer Greek yogurt, mixed berries, and chopped nuts in a glass or bowl.

2. Drizzle with honey if desired.

3. Serve immediately.

Cooking Time: Less than 5 minutes.

3. Overnight Chia Pudding

Prepare this easy and nutritious chia pudding the night before for a hassle-free breakfast.

Ingredients:

- 2 tbsp chia seeds
- 1/2 cup unsweetened almond milk
- 1/4 tsp vanilla extract
- 1/4 cup diced mango
- 1 tsp honey (optional)

Instructions:

1. Mix chia seeds, almond milk, and vanilla extract in a jar or bowl.

2. Cover and refrigerate overnight.

3. In the morning, top with diced mango and a drizzle of honey if desired.

4. Stir and enjoy.

Cooking Time: Overnight (about 8 hours).

4. Whole-Grain Oatmeal

A classic, hearty bowl of oatmeal made with whole grains and topped with your favorite fruits and nuts.

Ingredients:

- 1/2 cup rolled oats (whole grain)
- 1 cup water or unsweetened almond milk
- 1/4 cup sliced bananas
- 2 tbsp chopped almonds
- 1/2 tsp cinnamon

Instructions:

1. Cook oats with water or almond milk according to package instructions.

2. Top with sliced bananas, chopped almonds, and a sprinkle of cinnamon.

3. Serve warm.

Cooking Time: Approximately 5-7 minutes.

5. Avocado and Tomato Toast

This avocado and tomato toast is a satisfying, savory breakfast option that's low in carbohydrates.

Ingredients:

- 1 slice of whole-grain bread
- 1/4 ripe avocado
- 1 small tomato, sliced
- Salt and pepper to taste
- A dash of lemon juice

Instructions:

1. Toast the whole-grain bread.

2. Mash the ripe avocado and spread it on the toasted bread.

3. Top with sliced tomatoes, salt, pepper, and a dash of lemon juice.

4. Enjoy your open-faced sandwich.

Cooking Time: Approximately 5 minutes.

6. Peanut Butter and Banana Sandwich

A simple and filling sandwich that combines the creaminess of peanut butter with the natural sweetness of bananas.

Ingredients:

- 2 slices of whole-grain bread
- 2 tbsp natural peanut butter (no added sugar)
- 1/2 banana, sliced

Instructions:

1. Spread peanut butter on one slice of bread.

2. Top with sliced bananas.

3. Place the second slice of bread on top to make a sandwich.

4. Cut in half and serve.

Cooking Time: Less than 5 minutes.

7. Berry and Almond Smoothie

This berry and almond smoothie is a quick and convenient option for a nutritious breakfast on the go.

Ingredients:

- 1/2 cup unsweetened almond milk
- 1/2 cup mixed berries (e.g., strawberries, blueberries, raspberries)
- 1 tbsp almond butter (unsweetened)
- 1/2 tsp honey (optional)
- Ice cubes (optional)

Instructions:

1. Combine almond milk, mixed berries, almond butter, and honey (if using) in a blender.

2. Blend until smooth.

3. Add ice cubes if you prefer a colder consistency.

4. Pour into a glass and enjoy.

Cooking Time: Less than 5 minutes.

8. Scrambled Tofu with Spinach

A protein-rich and plant-based alternative to scrambled eggs, perfect for a satisfying breakfast.

Ingredients:

- 1/2 cup firm tofu, crumbled
- 1/4 cup chopped spinach
- 1/4 cup diced bell peppers
- 1/4 tsp turmeric (for color)
- Salt and pepper to taste
- 1 tsp olive oil

Instructions:

1. Heat olive oil in a pan over medium heat.

2. Add diced bell peppers and sauté until tender.

3. Add crumbled tofu, turmeric, salt, and pepper.

4. Cook until tofu is heated through and slightly crispy.

5. Stir in chopped spinach and cook until wilted.

6. Serve hot.

Cooking Time: Approximately 10 minutes.

9. Cottage Cheese with Berries

Cottage cheese provides a protein boost while mixed berries add natural sweetness and fiber.

Ingredients:

- 1/2 cup low-fat cottage cheese
- 1/4 cup mixed berries (e.g., blueberries, raspberries)
- 1 tsp honey (optional)

Instructions:

1. Spoon cottage cheese into a bowl.

2. Top with mixed berries and drizzle with honey if desired.

3. Enjoy this simple and satisfying breakfast.

Cooking Time: Less than 5 minutes.

10. Whole-Grain Waffle with Almond Butter

A whole-grain waffle topped with almond butter and banana slices is a tasty and filling way to start your day.

Ingredients:

- 1 whole-grain waffle (store-bought or homemade)
- 1 tbsp natural almond butter (no added sugar)
- 1/2 banana, sliced

Instructions:

1. Toast the whole-grain waffle.

2. Spread almond butter on the waffle.

3. Top with sliced banana.

4. Serve and enjoy your waffle sandwich.

Cooking Time: Approximately 5 minutes.

These breakfast recipes are designed to provide variety and nutrition while helping manage blood sugar levels for those newly diagnosed with diabetes. Remember to monitor portion sizes and adjust ingredients as needed based on your individual dietary requirements and preferences

Diabetes Diet Lunch Recipes for Newly Diagnosed

1. Grilled Chicken Salad

A light and satisfying salad with grilled chicken for lean protein.

Ingredients:

- 4 oz grilled chicken breast
- Mixed greens (e.g., spinach, arugula)
- Cherry tomatoes
- Cucumber slices
- Balsamic vinaigrette (low-sugar)

Instructions:

1. Season and grill chicken until cooked through.

2. Arrange mixed greens, cherry tomatoes, and cucumber on a plate.

3. Slice the grilled chicken and place it on top.

4. Drizzle with balsamic vinaigrette.

Cooking Time: Approximately 15 minutes (including grilling).

2. Lentil and Vegetable Soup

A hearty and fiber-rich soup that's perfect for lunch.

Ingredients:

- 1/2 cup dried green or brown lentils
- Mixed vegetables (e.g., carrots, celery, onions)
- Low-sodium vegetable broth
- Seasonings (e.g., thyme, bay leaves)
- Olive oil (optional)

Instructions:

1. Rinse lentils and set aside.

2. Sauté chopped vegetables in olive oil (if using) until softened.

3. Add lentils, vegetable broth, and seasonings.

4. Simmer until lentils are tender.

5. Serve hot.

Cooking Time: Approximately 30 minutes.

3. Turkey and Avocado Wrap

A satisfying wrap filled with lean protein and healthy fats.

Ingredients:

- Whole-grain wrap or tortilla
- Sliced turkey breast
- Avocado slices
- Lettuce
- Tomato slices
- Mustard (optional)

Instructions:

1. Lay out the wrap or tortilla.

2. Layer turkey slices, avocado, lettuce, and tomato.

3. Add mustard if desired.

4. Roll it up and cut in half.

Cooking Time: Less than 10 minutes.

4. Quinoa and Black Bean Salad

A protein-packed salad with quinoa and black beans for sustained energy.

Ingredients:

- Cooked quinoa
- Canned black beans (drained and rinsed)
- Chopped bell peppers
- Red onion, finely chopped
- Cilantro
- Lime vinaigrette dressing

Instructions:

1. Combine cooked quinoa, black beans, chopped bell peppers, red onion, and cilantro in a bowl.

2. Drizzle with lime vinaigrette dressing.

3. Toss to combine.

4. Serve chilled.

Cooking Time: Approximately 15 minutes (for quinoa preparation).

5. Tuna Salad Lettuce Wraps

A low-carb option featuring tuna salad in crisp lettuce cups.

Ingredients:

- Canned tuna in water (drained)
- Greek yogurt (unsweetened)
- Diced celery and red onion
- Dijon mustard
- Lettuce leaves

Instructions:

1. Mix tuna, Greek yogurt, celery, red onion, and Dijon mustard in a bowl.

2. Spoon the tuna salad onto lettuce leaves.

3. Roll the lettuce leaves to create wraps.

Cooking Time: Less than 10 minutes.

6. Chickpea and Vegetable Stir-Fry

A flavorful and fiber-rich stir-fry with chickpeas and colorful vegetables.

Ingredients:

- Cooked chickpeas
- Mixed vegetables (e.g., broccoli, bell peppers, snap peas)
- Low-sodium soy sauce
- Garlic and ginger (minced)
- Olive oil (optional)

Instructions:

1. Sauté minced garlic and ginger in olive oil (if using).

2. Add mixed vegetables and cooked chickpeas.

3. Stir-fry until vegetables are tender.

4. Drizzle with low-sodium soy sauce.

5. Serve hot.

Cooking Time: Approximately 20 minutes.

7. Spinach and Feta Stuffed Chicken Breast

A protein-rich and flavorful stuffed chicken breast.

Ingredients:

- Boneless, skinless chicken breast

- Fresh spinach leaves

- Feta cheese (reduced fat)

- Lemon juice

- Seasonings (e.g., oregano, garlic powder)

Instructions:

1. Preheat oven to 375°F (190°C).

2. Slice a pocket into each chicken breast.

3. Stuff with spinach, feta, and a sprinkle of lemon juice and seasonings.

4. Bake until chicken is cooked through.

Cooking Time: Approximately 25-30 minutes.

8. Lentil and Quinoa Bowl

A satisfying bowl filled with plant-based protein and fiber.

Ingredients:

- Cooked quinoa
- Cooked lentils
- Sautéed spinach and mushrooms
- Cherry tomatoes
- Balsamic vinaigrette (low-sugar)

Instructions:

1. Layer quinoa, lentils, sautéed spinach and mushrooms, and cherry tomatoes in a bowl.

2. Drizzle with balsamic vinaigrette.

3. Mix and enjoy.

Cooking Time: Approximately 25 minutes (including quinoa and lentil preparation).

9. Baked Salmon with Steamed Broccoli

A simple and heart-healthy lunch option featuring baked salmon.

Ingredients:

-   Salmon fillet
-   Lemon slices
-   Steamed broccoli
-   Olive oil
-   Seasonings (e.g., dill, garlic powder)

Instructions:

1. Preheat oven to 375°F (190°C).

2. Place salmon on a baking sheet, season with olive oil, lemon slices, and seasonings.

3. Bake until salmon flakes easily.

4. Serve with steamed broccoli.

Cooking Time: Approximately 20 minutes.

10. Turkey and Vegetable Stir-Fry

A lean and flavorful turkey stir-fry with assorted vegetables.

Ingredients:

- Ground turkey

- Mixed vegetables (e.g., bell peppers, snap peas, carrots)

- Low-sodium teriyaki sauce

- Garlic and ginger (minced)

- Olive oil (optional)

Instructions:

1. Brown ground turkey in a pan with olive oil (if using).

2. Add minced garlic and ginger.

3. Stir in mixed vegetables and teriyaki sauce.

4. Cook until vegetables are tender.

5. Serve hot.

Cooking Time: Approximately 20 minutes.

CHAPTER FOUR

Diabetes Diet Dinner Recipes for Newly Diagnosed

1. Baked Chicken and Vegetable Foil Packets

A simple and flavorful dinner option that requires minimal cleanup.

Ingredients:

- Chicken breast or thigh
- Sliced bell peppers
- Sliced zucchini
- Cherry tomatoes
- Olive oil
- Seasonings (e.g., Italian seasoning, garlic powder)

Instructions:

1. Preheat the oven to 375°F (190°C).

2. Place chicken and vegetables on a sheet of aluminum foil.

3. Drizzle with olive oil and season with desired seasonings.

4. Fold the foil into a packet and bake until the chicken is cooked through.

Cooking Time: Approximately 30 minutes.

2. Stir-Fried Tofu with Broccoli and Brown Rice

A plant-based, protein-rich dinner option with plenty of veggies.

Ingredients:

- Firm tofu, cubed
- Broccoli florets
- Low-sodium soy sauce
- Garlic and ginger (minced)
- Brown rice

Instructions:

1. Sauté minced garlic and ginger in a pan.

2. Add cubed tofu and brown until slightly crispy.

3. Stir in broccoli florets and low-sodium soy sauce.

4. Serve over cooked brown rice.

Cooking Time: Approximately 25 minutes (including rice preparation).

3. Grilled Salmon with Asparagus

A heart-healthy dinner featuring grilled salmon and asparagus.

Ingredients:

- Salmon fillet
- Asparagus spears
- Olive oil
- Lemon juice
- Seasonings (e.g., dill, garlic powder)

Instructions:

1. Preheat the grill to medium-high heat.

2. Season salmon with olive oil, lemon juice, and desired seasonings.

3. Place salmon and asparagus on the grill.

4. Grill until salmon flakes easily and asparagus is tender.

Cooking Time: Approximately 15-20 minutes.

4. Turkey and Quinoa Stuffed Peppers

A wholesome dinner with lean turkey and nutrient-rich quinoa.

Ingredients:

- Bell peppers
- Ground turkey
- Cooked quinoa
- Diced tomatoes (canned, low-sodium)
- Olive oil
- Seasonings (e.g., paprika, oregano)

Instructions:

1. Preheat the oven to 375°F (190°C).

2. Cut the tops off bell peppers and remove seeds.

3. Sauté ground turkey in olive oil until browned.

4. Mix cooked quinoa and diced tomatoes with turkey.

5. Stuff bell peppers with the mixture.

6. Bake until peppers are tender.

Cooking Time: Approximately 40 minutes (including baking).

5. Shrimp and Vegetable Stir-Fry

A quick and delicious stir-fry with shrimp and a medley of colorful vegetables.

Ingredients:

- Shrimp (peeled and deveined)
- Mixed vegetables (e.g., bell peppers, snap peas, broccoli)
- Low-sodium stir-fry sauce
- Garlic and ginger (minced)
- Brown rice

Instructions:

1. Sauté minced garlic and ginger in a pan.

2. Add shrimp and cook until pink and opaque.

3. Stir in mixed vegetables and low-sodium stir-fry sauce.

4. Serve over cooked brown rice.

Cooking Time: Approximately 20 minutes (including rice preparation).

6. Baked Cod with Spinach and Tomatoes

A light and flavorful dinner featuring baked cod with spinach and tomatoes.

Ingredients:

- Cod fillet
- Fresh spinach leaves
- Cherry tomatoes
- Olive oil
- Lemon juice
- Seasonings (e.g., basil, garlic powder)

Instructions:

1. Preheat the oven to 375°F (190°C).

2. Place cod on a baking sheet.

3. Drizzle with olive oil and lemon juice, then season with desired seasonings.

4. Top with spinach and cherry tomatoes.

5. Bake until the cod is cooked through.

Cooking Time: Approximately 20-25 minutes.

7. Eggplant and Chickpea Curry

A satisfying and fiber-rich curry with eggplant and chickpeas.

Ingredients:

- Eggplant, diced
- Canned chickpeas (drained and rinsed)
- Coconut milk (light)
- Curry paste (low-sodium)
- Olive oil
- Brown rice

Instructions:

1. Sauté diced eggplant in olive oil until softened.

2. Stir in chickpeas, coconut milk, and curry paste.

3. Simmer until eggplant is tender.

4. Serve over cooked brown rice.

Cooking Time: Approximately 30 minutes (including rice preparation).

8. Grilled Tofu and Vegetable Skewers

A plant-based dinner option with marinated tofu and colorful veggies.

Ingredients:

- Firm tofu, cubed
- Bell peppers, cherry tomatoes, zucchini (sliced)
- Marinade (low-sodium, e.g., balsamic vinaigrette)
- Wooden skewers (soaked)

Instructions:

1. Marinate tofu in the marinade for about 30 minutes.

2. Thread tofu and veggies onto soaked skewers.

3. Grill until tofu is lightly browned and veggies are tender.

Cooking Time: Approximately 15-20 minutes (including marinating and grilling).

9. Turkey and Vegetable Soup

A comforting and low-carb soup filled with turkey and vegetables.

Ingredients:

- Ground turkey
- Mixed vegetables (e.g., carrots, celery, green beans)
- Low-sodium chicken broth
- Seasonings (e.g., thyme, bay leaves)
- Olive oil (optional)

Instructions:

1. Brown ground turkey in a pot with olive oil (if using).

2. Add chopped vegetables and seasonings.

3. Pour in low-sodium chicken broth.

4. Simmer until vegetables are tender.

5. Serve hot.

Cooking Time: Approximately 30 minutes.

10. Spinach and Feta Stuffed Portobello Mushrooms

A vegetarian dinner option featuring savory stuffed portobello mushrooms.

Ingredients:

- Portobello mushrooms
- Fresh spinach leaves
- Feta cheese (reduced fat)
- Olive oil
- Seasonings (e.g., thyme, garlic powder)

Instructions:

1. Preheat the oven to 375°F (190°C).

2. Clean and remove the stems from portobello mushrooms.

3. Sauté fresh spinach in olive oil until wilted.

4. Stuff mushrooms with spinach and feta, then season with desired seasonings.

5. Bake until mushrooms are tender.

Cooking Time: Approximately 20-25 minutes.

Diabetes Diet Snack Recipes for Newly Diagnosed

1. Greek Yogurt and Berry Parfait

A protein-rich snack with the natural sweetness of berries.

Ingredients:

- 1/2 cup Greek yogurt (unsweetened)
- Mixed berries (e.g., strawberries, blueberries)
- 1 tbsp chopped nuts (e.g., almonds, walnuts)
- 1 tsp honey (optional)

Instructions:

1. Layer Greek yogurt, mixed berries, and chopped nuts in a glass or bowl.

2. Drizzle with honey if desired.

3. Serve immediately.

Preparation Time: Less than 5 minutes.

2. Sliced Cucumber with Hummus

A refreshing and crunchy snack with a protein-packed dip.

Ingredients:

- Sliced cucumber
- Hummus (low-fat and low-sodium)

Instructions:

1. Arrange cucumber slices on a plate.

2. Serve with a side of hummus for dipping.

3. Enjoy this satisfying and low-carb snack.

Preparation Time: Less than 5 minutes.

3. Mixed Nuts and Dried Fruit

A portable and balanced snack combining healthy fats and fiber.

Ingredients:

- A handful of mixed nuts (e.g., almonds, walnuts)
- A small portion of dried fruit (e.g., apricots, raisins)

Instructions:

1. Combine a variety of mixed nuts with a small portion of dried fruit in a snack-sized container.

2. This snack is perfect for when you're on the go.

Preparation Time: Less than 5 minutes.

4. Celery Sticks with Cream Cheese

A crunchy and creamy snack that's low in carbohydrates.

Ingredients:

- Celery sticks
- Low-fat cream cheese

Instructions:

1. Fill celery sticks with low-fat cream cheese.

2. Enjoy the satisfying contrast of textures and flavors.

Preparation Time: Less than 5 minutes.

5. Raw Bell Pepper Strips with Guacamole

A colorful and nutritious snack pairing fresh veggies with creamy guacamole.

Ingredients:

- Bell pepper strips (e.g., red, yellow, green)
- Guacamole (homemade or store-bought, low-sodium)

Instructions:

1. Arrange bell pepper strips on a plate.

2. Dip them in guacamole for a satisfying snack.

Preparation Time: Less than 5 minutes.

6. Cottage Cheese with Pineapple Chunks

A protein-packed snack with a hint of sweetness from pineapple.

Ingredients:

- 1/2 cup low-fat cottage cheese
- 1/4 cup pineapple chunks (fresh or canned in juice)

Instructions:

1. Spoon cottage cheese into a bowl.

2. Top with pineapple chunks.

3. Enjoy this balanced snack.

Preparation Time: Less than 5 minutes.

7. Apple Slices with a Sprinkle of Cinnamon

A simple and naturally sweet snack with a dash of flavor.

Ingredients:

- Apple slices
- Ground cinnamon

Instructions:

1. Slice an apple into thin rounds or wedges.

2. Sprinkle with ground cinnamon for extra flavor.

3. This snack is quick and satisfying.

Preparation Time: Less than 5 minutes.

8. Baby Carrots and Guacamole

A crunchy and creamy snack pairing baby carrots with guacamole.

Ingredients:

- Baby carrots
- Guacamole (low-sodium)

Instructions:

1. Serve baby carrots with a side of guacamole for dipping.

2. Enjoy the contrast of textures and flavors.

Preparation Time: Less than 5 minutes.

9. Sliced Pear with Almond Butter

A satisfying snack combining the sweetness of pear with the richness of almond butter.

Ingredients:

- Sliced pear
- Natural almond butter (no added sugar)

Instructions:

1. Slice a ripe pear into wedges.

2. Spread almond butter on each pear slice.

3. This snack is both satisfying and nutritious.

Preparation Time: Less than 5 minutes.

10. Plain Popcorn

A low-calorie and whole-grain snack that's perfect for satisfying your crunch cravings.

Ingredients:

- Popped plain popcorn (no butter or added salt)

Instructions:

1. Pop plain popcorn using an air popper or stovetop method.

2. Season with a sprinkle of herbs or spices for added flavor, if desired.

3. Enjoy this guilt-free snack.

Preparation Time: Varies depending on the popping method.

These snack recipes are designed to offer variety and nutrition while helping you manage blood sugar levels. Remember to adapt portion sizes and ingredients as needed to align with your dietary requirements and preferences.

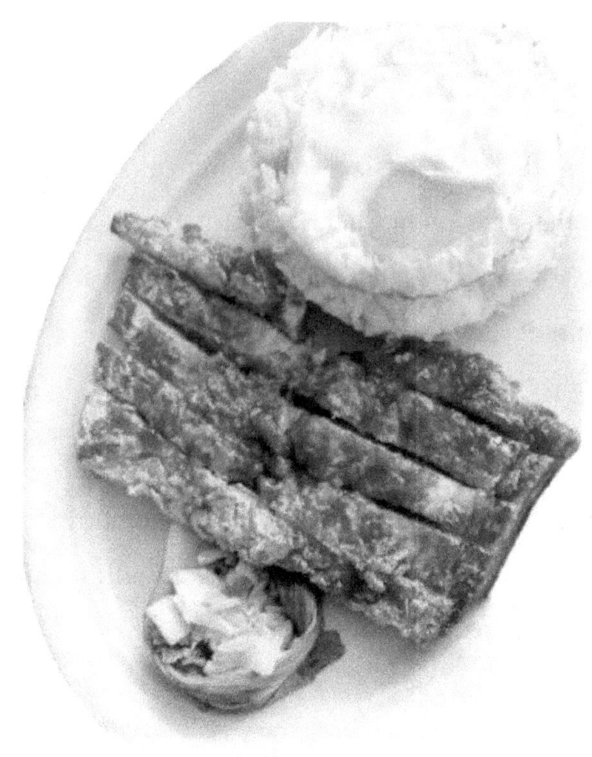

CONCLUSION

In conclusion, a diabetes diagnosis can be overwhelming, but with the right dietary approach and lifestyle changes, managing the condition becomes not only manageable but also an opportunity for improved overall health.

A well-balanced diabetes diet plays a pivotal role in stabilizing blood sugar levels, preventing complications, and enhancing one's quality of life.

The diabetes diet emphasizes choosing nutrient-dense, whole foods that are rich in fiber, lean proteins, healthy fats, and a variety of vitamins and minerals. Such a diet aids in regulating blood sugar levels and mitigating the risk of extreme highs and lows. It also helps with weight management, a crucial factor in diabetes control.

Key principles of a diabetes-friendly diet include portion control, carbohydrate management, and mindful eating. Portion control helps prevent overconsumption, which can lead to spikes in blood sugar.

Carbohydrate management involves monitoring and distributing carbohydrate intake throughout the day to maintain stable glucose levels. Mindful eating encourages individuals to be attuned to their hunger and fullness cues, fostering a healthier relationship with food.

A diabetes diet offers a diverse range of foods, allowing for flexibility and enjoyment in meal planning. Fresh vegetables, whole grains, lean proteins, and healthy fats can be combined to create delicious and satisfying meals. Additionally, incorporating regular physical activity and staying well-hydrated are essential components of diabetes management.

Ultimately, the goal of a diabetes diet is to provide the body with the necessary nutrients while preventing blood sugar spikes. However, it's important to remember that there is no one-size-fits-all approach to diabetes management.

Individualized care, including consultation with a registered dietitian or healthcare professional, is crucial to tailor the diet to one's unique needs and preferences.

In embracing a diabetes-friendly diet, individuals newly diagnosed with the condition can embark on a journey toward better health and improved blood sugar control.